Natural Crohns Disease Relief

How I Dealt With My Crohn's Disease Symptoms Successfully

May this book prove to you that it is actually possible to fight Crohn's disease, contrary to what the doctors may have said. It will give you hope that your diagnosis is not a life sentence.

A Shout Out To An Important Person That I Will Forever Thank

I'd like to thank Antony Muli for helping me bring this book to life. He has been instrumental in putting my disorganized story to life through his impeccable writing, editing, and formatting services.

Introduction

The year was 2017, and at 32 years of age, I was supposed to be at the peak of my physical health. However, the truth was that I had not been feeling well for a while. In fact, for the past 20 years of my life, I had experienced intermittent bouts of minor illnesses. I often chose to ignore the symptoms because things would always go back to normal after a while. However, this time was different; my symptoms continued to get worse. A fever, fatigue, and excruciating abdominal cramps had made my life a living hell. When I couldn't take the pain or stand up anymore, I checked myself into the emergency room. I didn't think much of it at the time, and I assumed I must have developed a common infection of some kind. I expected that some antibiotics would be all that I'd need, and I'd be on my way home. Unfortunately for me, the situation was much more serious than that. In fact, it was so dangerous that had I not checked myself into the hospital, I may never have gotten a chance to write this book at all.

It's been four years since I was admitted to the hospital, but I still remember my hospital room like I was there yesterday. Everything about that room, from the smell of the sheets to the color of curtains, is fresh as the day I left. I suppose that when you go through a major life-changing event, every detail about it tends to stick in your mind.

After spending four days in the hospital, I was getting impatient. The staff had been running a series of tests, and I wanted the results as quickly as possible. I remember the moment doctor Brown stepped into my room. From the expression on his face, I could see he was concerned. I wondered how terrible things must be as I braced myself for the bad news. He informed me that the lab results were back and that I had tested positive for Crohn's disease. I didn't understand what that meant, so he explained that it was a type of inflammatory bowel disease that affects the digestive tract. He then informed me that there was no cure for the disease and I would have to spend $5,000 per month to manage the symptoms.

I found this to be an unacceptable outcome, so I spent several months intensely researching the condition. Eventually, I came across Doctor Weston A. Price's ideas, which presented a unique approach that set me on a path to recovery. I am not a physician, and nothing in this book should be taken as medical advice. Nonetheless, this is my story of self-healing, and I hope you can learn from it.

Table of Contents

Introduction _____ 4

Chapter 1: My Experience _____ 8

Chapter 2: What is Crohn's Disease? _____ 14

    Understanding The Digestion Process _____ 15

    My Research into Crohn's Disease _____ 17

    Impact of Crohn's Disease on Quality of Life ___ 20

Chapter 3: Things to Avoid to Stop Injuring Your Gut _____ 22

    The Dangers of Eating at Fast Food Restaurants _____ 23

    Foods to Avoid _____ 27

Chapter 4: How to Kill the Infection _____ 50

    How to Use Oil of Oregano _____ 52

    Additional Reasons to Look After the Health of Your Gut _____ 56

Chapter 5: How to Heal Your Body _____ 58

Weston A. Price _____ 59

Exercise and Crohn's Disease _____ 61

Conclusion _____ 63

Thank You _____ 65

Chapter 1: My Experience

"Of pain, you could wish only one thing: that it should stop."

By George Orwell

Picture yourself at 12 years of age. Everything in life is exciting, new and it feels like nothing can hurt you. Playing outside and hanging out with friends is the highlight of your day and anything that gets in the way is nothing but an unwanted distraction. I was at this blissful and tender age when I first experienced the symptoms of my illness. Some mild abdominal discomfort that I took for nothing more than an annoyance that interfered with my daily pleasures.

It wasn't until I was in high school that my symptoms moved from being a petty vexation to a noticeable problem. I would experience several moments of abdominal pain, diarrhea, and a loss of appetite.

If there is one rule in high school, it's that your reputation is worth more to you than your life. Complaining about embarrassing symptoms like diarrhea could easily have made me a laughingstock, so I chose to keep my troubles to myself.

Even after I finished my education and got a job, I still chose to continue hiding my problems because they would often disappear after a while. I didn't know at the time that my stubbornness was going to cost me a lot of pain down the road.

The tipping point finally arrived in 2017 when my symptoms got considerably worse. I experienced a four-month period during which each day was more challenging than the one before. This time the symptoms weren't going away, and in fact, they were much worse than ever before. I remember how performing a simple task such as standing up had become near impossible. I would get up to fetch a glass of water, but before 30 seconds were up, I would start to feel dizzy. I would have blurred vision, my legs would get wobbly, a feeling of lightheadedness would overcome me, and eventually, I would lose my balance.

The day I finally decided to go to the hospital had been particularly tough. After arriving home from work, I hoped to get some rest, but I could feel my symptoms getting worse by the minute. I got in my car and drove myself to the hospital. After arriving, I walked into the ER and informed the nurse at the front desk that I was unwell and could barely stand. She requested a wheelchair on my behalf, and I got some mild reprieve as I sat down waiting to be treated. After about

15 minutes, the hospital staff took me into triage so they could perform an Electrocardiography (EKG). The purpose of the exam, as I would later come to learn, was to determine the health of my heart. The painless test worked by connecting a series of electrodes to specific areas of my chest to record the electrical signals coming from my heart. The doctors then collected some blood and asked a series of standard questions.

I was informed that given how busy the hospital was, I would have to wait for two hours for a room to open up in the ER. About 15-20 minutes later, two nurses walked into the waiting room, and it was clear to see from the worried expression on their faces that something was wrong. They informed me that I was anemic and then hurriedly rolled me out of the room on my wheelchair.

At this point, I had become genuinely scared, and I asked them what was going on. They seemed less concerned with answering my questions and more concerned about getting me to the ER. When we got there, I was shocked to see 6 staff members waiting for us. The second I was in the room, they took my shirt off, and I was asked to sign some legal paperwork. I could see two units of blood had been hooked up as I was injected with an 18 gauge IV needle into my left arm then a second 20 gauge IV needle into my right arm.

Anemia occurs when the body does not have enough red blood cells to carry much-needed oxygen throughout the body. The goal of the doctors was, therefore, to raise my red blood cells count as quickly as possible because they believed if my levels didn't rise immediately, then I was at risk of dying at any moment. I was informed that my situation was so bad that they had to redo the test two more times before they could believe the results.

The test revealed that my hemoglobin levels stood at 4.9 g/dL. To put this into context, the safe hemoglobin range for men is between 13.5 to 17.5 grams per deciliter, while for women, it's about 12.0 to 15.5 grams per deciliter. A 4.9g/dL level is considered dangerously low, and it explained why I was so fatigued and dizzy all the time. A litmus test was also performed, and it revealed the presence of blood in my rectum. In response, the doctors scheduled a colonoscopy and endoscopy to be conducted in two days' time so they could understand what was going on.

While I was alone in my bed, trying to mentally and emotionally process what was happening to me, 4 doctors suddenly broke into my room with a crash cart. They told me that my vital signs were crashing and they expected me to go into cardiac arrest at any moment. I felt fine so I actually made a joke that they were in the wrong room but I could see that nobody was interested in laughing. My heart rate averaged 188 beats per minute and my oxygen levels were abysmally low. Luckily I didn't go into cardiac arrest and my vital signs got back to normal.

A doctor eventually performed a colonoscopy and endoscopy exam. The test revealed that I had a severe case of Crohn's disease. In fact, it was so severe that the doctor stated that this was the worst ones he had ever come across. When your doctor makes a statement of that nature, it conveys to you the gravity of the situation, so I listened intently as he explained what Crohn's disease was and how it was causing the problems I was experiencing.

The doctor then recommended a drug that I would have to take for the rest of my life in order to mitigate the symptoms. He made it clear that Crohn's disease could not be treated by dietary changes or medicine. Calculating the monthly bill brought the costs to about $5,000, which would have made my life quite challenging. I decided that there must be a better way, so I decided to begin an in-depth phase of research into the nature of Crohn's disease so I could understand how to heal myself.

My research brought me a great deal of insights that set me on a path to healing. Today I am living a rich, fulfilled life free of pain and other terrible symptoms. Therefore, I have decided to share what I learned with the world because knowledge of this magnitude is meant to be shared.

Chapter 2: What is Crohn's Disease?

"Health is not valued until sickness comes."

By Thomas Fuller

If you walked into your doctor's office and asked him to define Crohn's disease, what would he tell you? The conventional medical view of Crohn's disease is that it's an inflammatory bowel disease (IBD) caused by the immune system attacking itself. Despite your doctor's best intentions, the definition he would give you would be completely wrong. This is the definition that I initially believed, but the more I dug deeper into this illness's nature, the more I was convinced that the mainstream view was completely wrong. From this original sin, doctors then prescribe medication that makes the situation worse, not better.

I understand that going against conventional wisdom is a bold gamble, but I would ask that you bear with me as I look to turn the topic of Crohn's disease on its head. To prove my hypotheses, I will provide you with a firsthand account of my experiences and new groundbreaking research that is questioning many of the precepts that have been accepted as fact by the medical community for decades.

In this chapter, I will provide you with an effective guide to understanding the nature of Crohn's disease because only by understanding the illness does it become possible to cure it.

Understanding The Digestion Process

Before I can get into my experience with Crohn's disease, it is first necessary to understand the nature of the digestive process. Once you have grasped how different parts of the gut work to keep you alive, it will be much easier to understand how things could go wrong and how this impacts your wellbeing.

The digestive system begins in the mouth and ends in the rectum. Its purpose is to ingest food, break it down, absorb nutrients and finally throw away unwanted material. This is a long and complex process involving several functions. It takes about six to eight hours for food to pass through the stomach and small intestines and about 36 hours for food to move through the colon.

Functions of The Stomach

This is the first stop that food makes after being consumed. Food goes from the mouth through the esophagus and into the stomach, where it stays for about 2 to 3 hours. The stomach serves three main functions. The first and most obvious is that the stomach stores food. The stomach can increase its volume capacity significantly while maintaining minimal internal pressure. This ensures that food only gradually passes to the next phase.

The second function is that the stomach contains significant levels of hydrochloric acid and enzymes that are designed to kill off unwanted foreign organisms such as bacteria and viruses. Finally is that the stomach helps in breaking down food into small digestible parts.

Functions of The Small Intestines

After food leaves the stomach, it passes into the small intestines through the pyloric sphincter in small pieces. The small intestines are very narrow but constitute the longest part of the digestive system at 22 feet. Working in conjunction with the liver and pancreas, the small intestines produce enzymes that further breakdown food into small parts. The entire length of the small intestines is covered in small finger-like projections called villi responsible for absorbing the nutrients in food. These nutrients are then shuttled into the bloodstream so they can keep your body functioning optimally.

Functions of The Large Intestines

The large intestines connect the small intestines to the rectum. Food enters the large intestines via the ileocecal valve for the final phase of digestion. Nearly all valuable nutrients have already been absorbed by the small intestines, and all that remains for the large intestines is the absorption of water, minerals, and salt. From here, all the indigestible materials are passed onto the rectum.

Now that you understand how your gut works, it is easy to understand why the disruptions caused by Crohn's disease can lead to malnutrition, weight loss, fatigue, and many other symptoms. When food cannot be adequately broken down and be absorbed, it becomes very difficult for the body to maintain normal functions.

My Research into Crohn's Disease

My first major break with traditional views on Crohn's disease is how the illness is perceived. The conventional view is that the disease is special or unique, but my research shows that this is not the case. Crohn's disease is, for the most part, similar to many other gut-related diseases that could all be classified as one illness. The only difference between Crohn's and other gut-related illnesses is that it is typically confined to the large intestines while the other diseases affect other parts of the digestive system.

Fungi and bad bacteria cause all these illnesses. The word 'bad' is used to differentiate bad bacteria - which are harmful

- from good bacteria, which the body needs. In the case of Crohn's disease, the name of the fungus is Candida. This is a genus of yeast that naturally occurs in the mouth and gut. In small amounts, it is perfectly normal, but in certain people, Candida can grow uncontrollably, which sets a chain reaction that results in what we refer to as Crohn's disease.

Researchers are now realizing that other variables such as stress, heredity, and a malfunctioning immune system are not the primary cause of Crohn's disease but mere risk factors that aggravate the illness. Interest is now shifting more heavily to candida as the principal cause of Crohn's disease.

Due to the misconception that the immune system is responsible for causing Crohn's disease, many doctors often recommend immunosuppressants as a treatment. This is a class of drugs designed to reduce the strength of the immune system. At a time when you should be focused on strengthening your immune system to fight the candida infection, the immunosuppressants make your system weaker. This is the worst possible treatment you could have, and it explains why there has been so little progress in the treatment of Crohn's disease.

The second primary cause of Crohn's disease is a bacterial infection known as Helicobacter pylori or H. Pylori in short.

This bacterial infection is primarily found in the stomach but can also be found in other regions of the gut. Ask any doctor, and they will tell you that H. Pylori is tough (but not impossible) to cure because of its notorious ability to develop a resistance to antibiotics. In fact, doctors often prescribe 2-3 different antibiotics, which are taken simultaneously in order to try and kill off the bacteria. Unfortunately, these drugs often fail to cure the problem because they don't address the root cause of H. Pylori.

Whether the cause is Candida or H. Pylori, both of these infections destroy the lining of the gut. The body senses the damage and sends out antibodies to fight the infection. This results in three critical effects that you need to understand. The first is that the sending of antibodies to fight the infection creates the illusion that the immune system is attacking itself and hence why many doctors believe this to be the case. Second is that conflict between antibodies and infection leads to inflammation which is a common symptom of Crohn's disease. Third is that the damage to the lining of the gut results in fever, diarrhea, pain, and headaches.

Impact of Crohn's Disease on Quality of Life

Living in constant pain plus the constant fear of trying to locate a bathroom can have several negative consequences on the quality of life of people living with Crohn's disease. One of the biggest implications of this disease is that it can cause depression in people living with it. Constantly living in pain combined with potentially embarrassing symptoms such as diarrhea and blood in the stool can be taxing on confidence and sense of self-esteem.

It's important to note that depression doesn't just come from embarrassing symptoms associated with Crohn's disease but is in fact directly linked to the illness itself. This is due to the hormone Serotonin, which is responsible for regulating mood and increasing a sense of happiness. Contrary to popular expectation, 90% of serotonin is actually produced in the stomach and not the brain. This means that poor gut health leads to inefficient production of this critical hormone which results in depression.

Another bad effect of Crohn's disease is that it can interfere with one's professional life. While I personally never missed a day of work because of Crohn's disease, I do believe that my efficiency could have been far greater if I had taken control of the situation sooner.

My personal relationships also took a hit because the fatigue meant I couldn't go out with friends, and it wasn't until I took control of my condition that I was able to discuss the issue openly.

Crohn's disease can also lead to a considerable dent in finances because of the various medicines required to manage the symptoms. Immunosuppressants to deal with inflammation, appetite stimulants to increase food intake, plus Imodium to deal with diarrhea are just a few of the many drugs that you may have to take. Collectively the cost can become a huge burden for you and your family.

Chapter 3: Things to Avoid to Stop Injuring Your Gut

"Although the world is full of suffering, it is also full of the overcoming of it."

By Helen Keller

Having swept aside the many fallacies associated with Crohn's disease, you now have a proper understanding of how the disease develops, what its symptoms are and why it is so misunderstood. The next phase of this book is to educate you on protecting your gut from further damage. What's great about this chapter is that even if you don't have Crohn's disease, you can gain a lot of insight into how to protect yourself from unwanted future problems.

Before proceeding any further, it is essential to note that the advice offered in this chapter should be followed to the letter. When you are attempting to improve your health or cure an illness there won't be much of a point to it unless you fully commit. If you remove 50% or even 70% of the foods damaging your gut, this will not be enough to eliminate all of your problems completely. You must strive towards achieving complete detachment from things that are harmful to your gut. As we proceed further, it will be clear why this is so important and why any compromise could negatively impact all aspects of your health.

The Dangers of Eating at Fast Food Restaurants

Rule number one to improving your dietary lifestyle is understanding that most of the food sold at your local grocery store is likely harming you. The only thing that could be worse is those trips you take to the fast-food restaurant. Trust me when I say that I understand the appeal of fast food both in terms of price and convenience, but this is simply something I had to give up for the sake of my health, and you will have to make the same choice I did.

So why is it such a bad idea to eat fast food? Well, there are so many reasons that I could write a whole book on this topic, but I will restrict myself to the most critical issues. The most commonly consumed meal at most fast food joints is French fries. To prepare them, restaurants use vegetable oil/canola oil which is categorized as a trans fat.

Trans fats are artificial fats created through a process of hydrogenation, which converts liquid fat into a semisolid state. The consumption of trans fat is associated with heart disease, diabetes, and strokes. This is not to say that all

French fries are killers. In fact, up until the '90s, most restaurants used pork lard/fat, which is considerably safer than the current alternatives. The shift to unhealthy materials was motivated by greedy individuals who took advantage of consumer ignorance.

So what is the connection between trans fat consumption and Crohn's disease? Researchers have been looking into this issue for a while. A 2015 study by D Aggarwal, H Burns found that 29% of people with Crohn's disease reported a significant worsening of symptoms resulting from eating unhealthy trans fats. It is believed that this is likely due to a lipid imbalance in people with Crohn's. Whatever the cause, what is important to note is that unhealthy fat should be the first thing to go from your diet. This means that you must read the ingredients section any time you use a new product to make sure there are no artificial fats added.

Note: One of the effects of Crohn's disease is weight loss. Some individuals with the illness may be tempted to try and recover this weight quickly through eating fast foods, but this would likely be counterproductive in the long run.

A second reason to avoid eating at fast-food restaurants is that most of their foods and beverages have artificial sweeteners, flavorings, and colorings. It's now common knowledge that these things are responsible for nervous system illnesses, depression, seizures, allergies, and fatigue. What is less understood is that these things are also responsible for worsening Crohn's disease. While researchers in the field long suspected this connection, the hypotheses received greater validity in 2018 when Case Western Reserve University's study was published. The study was conducted over six weeks, during which a group of individuals who have Crohn's disease was fed artificial sweeteners consistently. About 15% of those in the study reported a severe worsening of their symptoms in the form of blood in the stool, fatigue, and abdominal pain. The study found that the patients displayed a significant rise in unhealthy Proteobacteria in their gut.

Did you know that the average bottle of coke has 12 teaspoons of sugar and a can of Pepsi has about seven teaspoons? The odds are high that you likely consume one of these two drinks when you make a stop at a fast-food restaurant. Sugar accelerates tooth decay, heart disease, and diabetes. This is all common knowledge, but what is less known is that because companies know that consumers understand how dangerous sugar is, they have created over 61 different names for sugar to camouflage this fact from their unsuspecting consumers. It almost feels like these companies are out to kill us, and if one doesn't stay sharp, they will likely succeed.

Many edible products in your home most likely contain sugar, even if the wording isn't written on the packaging. With this knowledge in mind, I decided that there was only one solution to this problem: to take control of as much of the cooking process as possible. As the old saying goes, *if you want something done right, do it yourself.*

Hygiene is also a critical factor that you need to keep in mind about eating at fast-food restaurants. This is because these places are trying to prepare as many meals as possible and don't really care about you as an individual. Therefore, they may take shortcuts in preparing your meal or be careless about the cooking area's level of cleanliness. It's very easy for bacterial, viral, and fungal infections to be served up in your food, which will later be a source of problems for your gut.

The final thing to take note of about eating out is that you may have noticed that the bread served at many fast-food restaurants appears to be alluringly white. This white color is designed to be attractive but is quite dangerous to your health. The chemical agents used to create this white effect should be avoided at all costs due to its damage to the gut.

Let us now look at the foods you should not eat:

Foods to Avoid

I'm going to present you with a list of foods you will need to learn to avoid, like the plague. These foods either weaken your gut or are responsible for encouraging infections in you. These foods include:

Orange juice

Despite its popularity, orange juice is one of the many fake health foods out there, causing a lot of damage to people's health and in particular, the gut. So why are fake health foods so dangerous? Because when people believe they are consuming something healthy but it isn't, they will take a lot of it, thinking they are helping themselves when they are only making things worse. It's very common for friends and relatives to bring orange juice to people recovering from an illness, but this is never a good idea.

Orange juice contains artificial sugars which are pasteurized at temperatures of 160F-200F. Sugar is unnaturally unhealthy, but this process makes things even worse because it destroys the vitamins and other nutrients contained within them.

Patsy Catsos is a health expert based in Portland. She notes that even if the sugar contained is natural, as in the case of raw fruit juice, it would still be better to take water over orange juice. High sugar content, she notes, always leads to a worsening of symptoms. To illustrate how dangerous orange juice can be, I will point out that an average glass of orange juice contains about 8 oranges worth of sugar water with zero fiber.

Grocery store bread

Bread is a high source of carbs which can be a good thing. It's a commonly held belief that carbs are bad, but this is not necessarily the case. While homemade bread could be healthy for you, it is best to avoid grocery store bread because of the preservatives, coloring, and other chemicals they add for commercial purposes. Even if the bread is whole grain in nature, this does not make it any better. This is because many commercial bakers use bleaching chemicals that are capable of killing off good bacteria in the gut.

There is a common misconception that whole grain is the healthy option, and many commercial bakers market their products along this lie. The truth is that whole grain bread is just as bad because it is made using seed coating. This coating cannot be properly digested and contains harmful compounds that were meant to protect the seed.

It's important to note that it's common practice for commercial bakers to use high fructose syrup to add taste to their products as well as chemical agents to stop their bread from going stale. When baking for yourself, you have the option of using a healthier alternative in the form of low amounts of natural sugar which can achieve the same intended effect. This is because natural sugar molecules have hygroscopic properties, which allow them to grab and hold moisture. Baked products made with natural sugar last longer than those without it.

Grain-fed red beef

Many people picking meat for their families aren't aware that the meat can be categorized into two categories. These categories are either grain or grass-fed. The names emerge from whether the cow was fed grass or grain. In the past, cows roamed and ate grass, but today many cows eat grain that has been grown by humans. These two different food sources significantly impact the nutritional composition of the beef that will later be consumed.

When it comes to diet, a rule of thumb is that you should always stick as close as possible to what is natural and avoid that which is artificial. Farmers prefer to feed their cows artificially grown grain because it is cheap, and it results in cow meat that is tenderer than grass-fed meat. Unfortunately, this advantage is a double-edged sword because cows did not evolve to eat grain but grass. The grass-fed meat contains more than five times the amount of Omega 3 fatty acids and twice conjugated linoleic acid (CLA). These compounds are helpful in avoiding heart disease, fighting diabetes, and building up healthy cholesterol. It's also important to note that grain-fed meat has antibiotics that kill off beneficial bacteria in the gut, unlike grass-fed meat.

Grass-fed meat also contains higher levels of vitamin A, which is good for helping internal organs function properly, and vitamin E, which is an antioxidant responsible for protecting cells from damage caused by free radicals.

Despite all the positive benefits to grass-fed meat that have been mentioned above, it is important to note that a lot of meat that has been labeled as grass fed may actually still be partially grain-fed. By keeping consumption below 20%, the meat can still be classified as grass-fed, even though this is not the case. Equally important is that the quality of the meat is radically impacted by how nutritious the grass that was fed to the cow. The quality of the grass is itself affected by the quality of the soil it grows in. The more diverse and abundant the soil biology is, the more nutritional the grass will be. This will lead to a healthier cow, and you, in turn, will receive more nutritional value per pound of meat at far lower calorie levels.

Some farmers give their cattle synthetic compounds and growth hormones such as estrogen, progesterone, and testosterone. There is growing public awareness about the dangers of these chemicals, so I won't dwell much on this topic other than to state that this often leads to mastitis, which is an inflammation of the breasts that requires heavy use of antibiotics.

So what is the solution to the meat problem? I bet you do not have a backyard big enough to grow enough grass to feed a cow, so I recommend visiting various grocery shops until you find one that is selling grass-fed meat that's free of antibiotics and growth hormones.

Non-Pastured Chicken

Many people buy chicken because it is a tasty yet affordable protein source, and most people fail to ask why the chicken is so cheap in the first place. Unfortunately, the answer to this question is not a pleasant one. The practices adopted by various farmers when rearing chicken are responsible for creating meat not suitable for human consumption. The chickens are housed in cramped quarters where the likelihood of getting an infection is very high. To counter this problem, farmers give their chicken antibiotics, which can be hazardous to humans.

Many factory-farmed chickens are fed a diet of soy. This soy mimics estrogen in the human body resulting in weight gain in men as well as erectile dysfunction (ED) and low testosterone.

Fruits

This one probably comes as a surprise, given that every health website out there recommends eating fruits as healthy. I am not saying that they are wrong; in fact, fruits contain essential nutrients that enhance the body's immune system. Unfortunately you have to be a little careful about your fruit consumption both in terms of quality and quantity. There are several reasons for this, and I will explain them below.

The first thing to understand is that while artificial sugars are quite dangerous, natural sugars aren't perfect either. Natural sugar sources like fruits, when overly consumed, can disrupt the intestinal mucus barrier, which will cause a worsening of symptoms. Equally important is that natural sugar messes up your insulin and thyroid sensitivity.

A second reason fruits are a problem is that they contain a high amount of insoluble fiber. This is an issue that I haven't discussed yet, but it is very critical. When suffering from Crohn's disease, the bowels can become narrow, and the linings can be significantly damaged. This means that when you consume insoluble fiber, this material can cause further damage to the digestive system or, worse, cause a blockage in the intestinal tract. A blocked tract is something that quickly becomes a life-threatening condition.

Fruits that contain insoluble fibers include kiwi, rhubarb, raspberries, strawberries, pineapple, grapes, and raisins.

It's also important to make sure that you source your foods from farmers who do not use chemicals in growing their food. For example, bananas are wrapped in a plastic bag when growing to protect them from pests. Unfortunately, this bag is sprayed with pesticides that come into contact with the banana, which you will eventually eat.

Vegetables

Just like fruits, this one must seem strange as well. But just as in the case of fruits, certain vegetables contain a high level of insoluble fiber that can be hazardous to your health. Beans, green peas, spinach, and zucchini are a few examples of vegetables with insoluble fiber.

There is another reason to be cautious about over-consuming vegetables, and this has to do with how they are grown. If the natural balance of the bacteria or fungus in the soil growing the vegetables has been destroyed, then this can result in vegetables that are not ideal for your gut

You might say that this is worth the risk because as everyone knows, vegetables are the richest source of vitamins. However, this misconception is why so many health experts overly emphasize the consumption of vegetables without weighing in certain critical variables into the equation. Yes, vegetables indeed contain essential vitamins, but their richness has been affected by human intervention over the years. For example, the use of salt-based fertilizers by farmers can lead to an accumulation of chlorine, boron, and sodium in plant leaves and stems, causing unhealthy plants in terms of nutritional value. A big misconception is that you get a lot of vitamins from vegetables. There are vitamins and minerals in vegetables but they are not as easily available and absorbed by the body as animal based vitamins and minerals are. It is commonly thought that you get a lot of vitamin A from carrots. That is false. Carrots contain beta-carotene. The body still needs to convert this into a usable form for the human body which is called retinol or the animal form of vitamin A. You also need the presence of fat for the body to be able to absorb it. If you ate a raw carrot only about 3% of the beta-carotene would be converted into retinol. Cooking the carrots would increase this slightly but still not an efficient way to provide vitamin A for the body. Many vegetables are sprayed with chemical fertilizers and pesticides. Vegetables that are produced in the ground like carrots and potatoes are especially at risk when fertilizers and pesticides are used. Eat vegetables in moderation like everything else. They contain health benefits but can also have many harmful effects if consumed in excess or from poor farming practices.

For example, let us look at tomatoes. Tomatoes are technically fruits, but for various reasons, nutritionists count them as vegetables. Naturally grown tomatoes are rich in Vitamin C, folic, and potassium, but unfortunately, human intervention has created unhealthy tomatoes. When tomatoes are picked from the farm, they are still green. This is done to make them easier to transport without damaging them. Unfortunately, once they have reached their target destination, it suddenly becomes a financial liability to physically house them until they can naturally turn red through ripening. To hasten the process, farmers use a chemical called ethylene in its gaseous state. When consumed, these tomatoes can cause stomach upsets and even diarrhea. Another problem is that ethylene turns the tomato red on the outside without actually ripening it on the inside. So the taste of the tomato isn't all that great either.

Have you ever wondered why fruits turn from green to different colors as they ripen? When fruits are unripe, they contain a chemical called chlorophylls which accounts for their green color. As they ripen, they lose this chemical. This happens to signal to plants the fruit is ready for consumption because the seeds are fully matured. Before this point the fruits contains a lot of anti-nutrients and is not ideal for your gut.

Non-Organic Foods

Non-organic food is grown using chemicals, fertilizers, and genetic enhancements to increase productivity, quantity and fight off disease. Despite the positive attributes created by the use of chemicals, there are also negative consequences. This is why many people have been shifting to buying foods labeled as organic at the grocery store.

While this is indeed a positive development, it should be noted that there is more to the story for individuals with Crohn's disease than chemical use. To make my point, I will reference the work of Dr. Elaine Ingham, one of the world's most respected microbiologist and soil expert. She is the author of the Soil Biology Primer used by the United States Department of Agriculture (USDA). In 2015, she gave a speech to the Oxford Real Farming Conference that left many of the attendees in awe for its startling revelations. She insisted that soil health was the key to creating nutritious, healthy plants. More important than this is that she showed that the connection between soil bacteria and gut health *"is not mere rhetoric but an evolutionary truth."*

The health of plants depends on the biodiversity of the fungus and bacteria in the soil. The higher the level of good bacteria and fungus in the soil the higher the mineral and vitamin content will be in the plants and hence healthier for us. Dr. Ingham research showed that by simply altering soil biology plants can increase the protein concentration in grass from 4% to 24%. Which cow do you think is healthier, the one eating 4% protein grass or 24% protein grass?

Something else to watch out for is genetically modified foods. GMOs are designed to be resistant to pests. This is achieved by giving the plants a toxin called *Bacillus thuringiensis* or simply BT. When this toxin is ingested by pests, it is activated by the high PH level in the gut of the insect. BT destroys the integrity of the gut lining, causing the insect's stomach to be destroyed. It was believed that BT toxin in such low amounts was harmless to humans, but research is showing that it simply takes longer for the adverse effects to show themselves.

Water Flavorings

This is something else that is advertised as healthy, which is actually the exact opposite. The water often has high levels of acidity that can be harmful to your gut. The artificial sweeteners, flavorings, and color are a combination of chemicals that could further inflame your gut. A few of the names of these common fake sugars are Aspartame, Neotame, Saccharin, and Sucralose. These fake sugars destroy your good fungus and bacteria.

A1 Milk

Milk can be categorized into two main groups depending on the origin of the cows that produced it. A1 milk is produced by cows that lived in European regions, while A2 milk comes from cows that lived on the Indian subcontinent. A1 cows produce far more milk than A2 cows, which is why commercial milk producers prefer it. Unfortunately, A1 milk contains proteins that are harmful to the gut. This problem is not found with raw A2 milk, and I can personally attest to this fact. I used to believe I was lactose intolerant, but I have personally drunk an 8 oz glass of raw A2 milk with every meal I have eaten for the last two years with no issues.

Pasteurized Milk

I will make a bold statement and say that there is no such thing as lactose intolerance. Yes, you read that right. The idea that certain people are incapable of digesting lactose is the result of a misunderstanding of the condition. When milk goes undergoes pasteurization, it loses the essential enzymes that would help in the digestive process. This is because enzymes are proteins and heat denatures protein. In fact, the test for successful pasteurization is the absence of all enzymes.

Luckily there is a small but growing number of researchers who realize that pasteurization is largely responsible for the lactose intolerance problem. A 2014 study of Maryland residents found that 59 of 153 individuals experienced discomfort after drinking pasteurized milk but zero discomfort after drinking raw unpasteurized milk. Raw milk also contains micro and macronutrients of vital importance to the human body. The minerals and vitamins in milk may not be too high, but they are 100% absorbed by the body. The fungus and bacteria responsible for Crohn's disease are already present in everyone's digestive system. They only become hazardous once we engage in activities that create an imbalance within the system. An example of this would be consuming antibiotics that kills bacteria in the gut, thus allowing the fungus to grow wildly out of control.

Throughout most of our history, humans drank milk in its raw form. Our bodies evolved with the knowledge that milk contains the necessary enzymes required for its digestion. Then came the French scientist Lois Pasteur, who in the 1860's, demonstrated the process of pasteurization. Pasteurization kills the necessary healthy bacteria needed to digest milk

Table salt

Most salt sold at the grocery store is 97 percent or more sodium chloride. There is usually a chemical anticaking agent mixed in as well. Consuming this salt can lead to many health problems, including high blood pressure and heart disease. Switch to using a natural sea salt. Pink himilyian can be good as well but depending on the brand could contain impurities that you do not want to consume.

Pain Relievers

Crohn's disease can result in chronic abdominal pain. It is tempting to simply rush to the drug store and buy the first pain relief medicine you can find, but this can be a very dangerous idea. Non-steroidal anti-inflammatory drugs (NSAIDs) such as Motrin (ibuprofen) or Aleve (naproxen)

are known to worsen Crohn's disease. Tylenol (acetaminophen), for example, is known to be a much safer alternative to the drugs mentioned above. In principle, however, you should simply stay away from all pain relief medicine whenever possible. The more you use them, the more dependent you become on them and resulting in the degradation of your joints.

The best way to ensure you don't have to use drugs is to eat a balanced nutritious diet coupled with engaging in exercise to strengthen your body overall.

Artificial Multivitamins

The consumption of multivitamin pills is not necessarily a bad thing and can, in fact, be beneficial. However, the problem is that people who take them tend to ignore the necessity of eating a balanced diet because they assume that they are getting everything they need. There is also a lack of clarity regarding the alleged benefits that are written on the bottles. For example, simply stating Vitamin D does not differentiate between vitamin D2 and Vitamin D3. Many of the vitamins added to the multivitamins are manmade. They do not have the same benefit as the vitamins you get from consuming real food.

Probiotic Pills

Probiotics are bacteria and yeast that live in your gut and serve a beneficial purpose. Pharmaceutical companies sell probiotic pills to people hoping to improve the quality of their digestion. While this may sound good in theory, the truth is that it is not the most efficient way to accomplish the intended objective. The reason these pills are ineffective is that before they can reach the small and large intestines, they are already burned out by the acid contained in the stomach. The PH level of stomach acid ranges between 3 to 1. To put this into context, the acidity level of acid in your car battery is 0, which means that your stomach is almost as acidic as a car battery. This is how food is broken down so effectively before advancing further, but so are the probiotic pills.

The best way to improve the probiotic levels in your gut is to eat foods that can naturally improve good bacteria. Yogurt, kombucha, sauerkraut, miso, kimchi and kefir are great examples.

Soy Products

There was a lot of buzz in 2017 after Researchers from Pennsylvania State University declared that their research revealed that soy products could alleviate symptoms associated with Crohn's disease, such as bowel inflammation and the loss of gut barrier function. This has led to an increase in the number of people consuming soy products. This is a mistake because, despite the purported benefits of soy consumption, there are downsides that make this a double-edged sword.

It's been known for decades that soy results in hormonal imbalances in both men and women. Further, research has revealed just how severe this problem is. Soy consumption leading to an excess of estrogen in women has been linked to breast cancer and bloating, decreased sex drive, irregular periods, mood swings, headaches, weight gain, and even hair loss. In men consuming large amounts of soy can reduce the amount of testosterone present in their bodies, leading to ED, male breasts, muscle loss and weight gain. Originally soy sauce was fermented for a minimum of two years before it was consumed.

Yogurt

In an earlier section, yogurt was presented as a great source of probiotics; it may therefore seem strange that it is also listed as a potentially hazardous food. The positive or negative effects of yogurt depend entirely on where you acquire it. Nearly all the yogurt sold at local grocery shops either has an excess of sugar or has been prepared in a manner that kills the healthy bacteria that you need.

Condiments

Condiments are spices and sauces added to food after it has been cooked to improve flavor. Understandably, we should want to make our food as tasty as possible, and I would not say that you should eliminate all condiments from your diet. However, it is important to note that most of the commercially sold condiments that you find at the grocery store contain high amounts of sugar for taste, artificial color to be alluring, and preservatives so they can last long on the shelves. All these additives will damage your gut and should be avoided at all costs.

Strange as it may sound, it is very easy to make homemade condiments that will not only be healthy but far tastier. Commercially processed condiments are mass-produced without the special type of care that an individual would have at home. I was very surprised at how much the quality of my food improved by taking the bold step of controlling my diet and what goes into my body. Trust me on this issue, and you will find that it is worth the effort.

Here is an example of a recipe that you can try out for yourself;

Recipe for 1 cup of mayonnaise

Ingredients

2 large eggs pastured raised soy free

2 teaspoons of freshly squeezed lemon

1 cup of neutral-flavored olive oil

1 pinch of salt

Method of preparation

Step 1: Separate egg whites from yolks and pour yolks into a bowl.

Step 2: Add the lemon juice into the bowl and stir.

Step 3: Gradually add the oil as you stir until it thickens.

Step 4: If the mayonnaise becomes too thick, add some water.

Step 5: Add a pinch of salt as you stir.

Step 6: Add spices of your choosing like paprika, vinegar, garlic, and onion.

Step 7: Pour a glass ready to serve

None of the ingredients mentioned here contain an ounce of processed chemicals or preservatives, yet the quality is superior. There are many other recipes that could fill an entire book, such as natural Ketchup, wasabi, and fish sauce, just to name a few.

Factory-Farmed Eggs

One of the best decisions you could ever make in life is to start eating pastured eggs. This is because they are full of essential nutrients and good cholesterol. Grocery store eggs have labels on the packaging that are very misleading. Cage free does not mean the chicken was allowed to move around because there are no spacing requirements. You are most likely over paying for your factory farmed eggs with a fancy misleading label on it at the grocery store.

Factory eggs are not as nutritious because the nutrition contained in the yolk of an egg comes directly from the hen. If the hen is fed cheap synthetic foods of soy, then the egg's quality will be equally bad.

To get the best eggs, you should source them from a local farm where you can confirm that the hens are actually fed a natural diet free of soy and gmo.

Store-bought Butter

Like with milk, the cow's quality determines whether the butter you consume is healthy or not. The butter should come from grass-fed cattle. Butter that comes from raw milk during the summer months when the grass is growing the fastest will have the highest amount of vitamin k2, which many people are deficient in. Vitamin K2 has been shown to decrease tooth decay and heart disease, promote calcification of bones while preventing the calcification of blood vessels and kidneys. Pasteurization by high heat also kills off vitamins and minerals that are key for our health

Grocery Store Bacon

Bacon has a bad reputation due to the fat it contains however, it is essential to note that bacon, which contains natural saturated fat, can actually be healthy. Saturated fat from a healthy animal will provide nutrition, keep you satiated and help you lose weight. Yes, natural saturated fat will help you actually lose weight. The unhealthy aspect is not the fat but the nitrate preservatives and the sugar that is added to grocery store bacon.

Coffee

There are worse things for you than coffee. Caffeine really could be considered a poison to the body but again there are worse things for you. The big problem with coffee is what everyone adds to it; excessive sugar, fake creamer, artificial caramel flavoring.

Antacids

It is essential to avoid antacids as much as possible since they are a temporary fix that causes long-term damage to the gut. The lower esophageal sphincter (LES) is a muscle that connects the stomach and the esophagus. It is responsible for preventing acid from leaving the stomach, and it does this by measuring PH levels.

When an antacid is taken, it raises the pH of the stomach acid (making it more alkaline), causing the pain to go away temporarily but also, over time, increasing the pH of the stomach acid so the muscle stops working and won't stay closed. Bad bacteria also do not like the acidic environment of your stomach, so they will create alkaline chemicals to raise the pH of your stomach acid to help them survive better. You need to make sure to kill off any bad bacteria and fungus and then start to rebuild the acidity of your stomach acid. This can be done with HCL supplements, sips of apple cider vinegar, ginger, and fermented vegetables like kimchi, sauerkraut, kefir and raw milk yogurt. The good bacteria will help your body correct the pH of your stomach acid. Not having a low enough pH of your stomach acid also leads to food not being completed digested. Excess fat stored on the stomach can also cause acid reflux. As you begin to heal and eat a more nutritious diet, you will very slowly begin to lose weight. A normal stomach acid level also ensures that all of your food is being broken down properly in the stomach and not being fermented inside of the intestines. Chewing food completely can also help reduce acid reflux. If you are a fast eater, you should try slowing down and taking a few more bites before you swallow.

Now that you understand how certain foods can negatively impact your gut's health, the next step is figuring out what you need to do to eliminate the infection that already exists. The fourth chapter will help you do just that.

Chapter 4: How to Kill the Infection

"To be prepared is half the victory."

By Miguel de Cervantes

According to several mainstream medical practitioners, it is essentially impossible to kill Crohn's infection deliberately. In instances where this does happen, it is simply labeled as a matter of luck. Therefore, they prescribe expensive medicines to help you manage the symptoms rather than getting cured. This chapter is about helping you understand how you can consciously take control of your life to kill the infection.

Before proceeding any further, I would like to point out that successfully killing the infection varies in difficulty depending on its severity. The location of the infection within the digestive tract and the severity of the damage it has inflicted are critical in determining how easy the process of killing the infection will be.

At this stage, you may be wondering why you should be listening to my advice at all?

To answer this question, I will state that the severity of my illness and the pain it caused me made me highly motivated to find a solution to my problem. I spent countless hours and thousands of dollars trying different products purported to kill infections in the gut. Like a medieval sorceress trying to find the elixir of life, I scoured the far reaches of the internet to try and find a solution to my problems. Over time, I developed a comprehensive understanding of what solutions work from the fake ones. The knowledge I acquired over this time will be a cheat code for you to help prevent you from wasting precious time with solutions that will never work.

An example of an idea that I experimented with was fasting. Several charlatans claim that radically reducing food consumed over 30 days will starve the harmful bacteria and fungus, thus leaving your gut free and clear.

Despite my effort, the process of starving myself out only resulted in weight loss with little to show for it. It took further study to understand that bacterial and fungal infection can survive in the gut for a long time, even with the drastic reduction in food consumption. They simply adapt by feeding on intestinal walls instead of the regular food that was being consumed. This is not to say that fasting does not have beneficial effects. As you will see in a later chapter, fasting can play an essential role in cell repair during healing, but it cannot kill the infection.

After my failed experiment, I eventually came across something that positively impacted my gut infection. This remedy effectively eliminates fungal and bacterial infections, which is why I consider it the most impressive solution to eliminating Crohn's disease infections. The pleasant secret that saved my life was consuming oil of oregano.

How to Use Oil of Oregano

Oil of oregano can either be consumed as a liquid or in pill form. When using the oil in a liquid form, your primary goal is to preserve the natural nutritional value as much as possible. Buy cold-pressed organic oil of oregano. The best time to consume this is half-way through your first meal of the day. To achieve this, follow the step below;

Step 1: Prepare a small amount of organic coconut oil

Step 2: Warm it slightly

Step 3: Add oil of oregano to it (because of different concentrations and purity it's impossible to give an exact ratio)

Step 4: Stir to mix

Step 5: Consume

It may be tempting to consume more oil of oregano, but this would be a mistake. First, is that consuming more oil of oregano will not lead to the killing of the infection faster Secondly, even if it were possible to kill off the infection quicker, the outcome would likely be negative. The process of destroying fungus candida tends to generate harmful toxins entering your bloodstream. These toxins result in flu-like symptoms, but if the accumulation is too great and can't be filtered out quickly enough, you could be at the risk of death.

This risk of death is low, but it can be mitigated even further by using activated charcoal when you are using oregano oil. Toxins in the human body are filtered out through the liver. The liver achieves this by using low-pressure vascular channels called sinusoids. These channels are lined with immune cells called Kuppfer. These cells are designed to identify foreign entities, engulf them and finally excrete them. This process is called phagocytosis, and despite being quite effective, it can be made better by the use of activated charcoal. This compound can trap toxins and chemicals in the gut before they are even absorbed. It is so effective that it is used in liver dialysis when a person has severe liver failure. Activated charcoal is great for the gut because it can judiciously distinguish between good and bad bacteria. I can personally attest to the fact that in the moments when I failed to consume the activated charcoal, I would feel terrible across my entire body because of the accumulation of toxins. However, please note that you should use activated charcoal in moderation for safety reasons.

As already stated earlier, the liquid form isn't the only way to consume oregano oil because pills also do the job just as well. In fact, I prefer consuming pills to liquid not just because it's more efficient this way but also because the pill contains other essential nutrients that help fight the infection. Examples of these helpful additives include herbal cleanser that promotes balance within the large and small intestines. A combination of protease, cellulose, and Aloe Vera helps promote proper cellular functions and improve the gut's lining. My brand of choice is a product from 1md.org called BalanceMD. This drug has been instrumental in helping turn my life around. It's important to note that you will start to feel better soon after you begin taking the drug but do not relent in the process. The road to recovery is a long one, and just because the symptoms have abated doesn't mean that you should take a lax attitude.

There are a few other things you could be doing to improve the quality of your gut. Certain foods can naturally help in the killing of bacterial and fungal infections in the gut. Here are a couple of examples;

Raw Honey

This is a fantastic superfood that simultaneously attacks fungal, bacterial, and viral infections. This is because it naturally contains hydrogen peroxide, which is an antiseptic.

This is why hospitals used to use it to treat open wounds. Honey also has a few additional benefits to your body, namely;

- It is a natural antioxidant

- It is a phytonutrient powerhouse that helps fight infections

- It kills H. Pylori that is responsible for stomach ulcers

- Soothe a sore throat

- It nourishes good gut bacteria

Apple Cider Vinegar

ACV has been used for a wide range of purposes in the home for centuries. It has been used as a home cleaning agent as well as a natural deodorant.

Apple cider vinegar is created by crushing apples into yeast, which ferments the sugar to turn it into alcohol. Bacteria are added to ferment the alcohol further until it turns into acetic acid. Organic unfiltered vinegar consists of a substance referred to simply as mother, and it contains enzymes, proteins, and friendly bacteria.

Apple cider vinegar is highly effective at killing off harmful bacteria while strengthening good bacteria. It also simultaneously helps with fighting diabetes and improving blood sugar levels.

Yogurt

The right kind of yogurt can be your greatest ally when it comes to improving the quality of bacteria in the gut. Ensure that it is as close to natural as possible and be free of preservatives, sugar, and artificial flavorings.

Additional Reasons to Look After the Health of Your Gut

Poor gut health has been linked to several other problems that at first may appear unrelated but should be taken seriously. Strange as it may sound, about 70% of your body's immune defenses are centered around your gut.

For example, the healthy bacteria in the gut help the stimulation of T-cells that are responsible for helping your body differentiate between harmful foreign entities in the body and regular tissue and cells.

Also, the vagus nerve is a critical nerve that travels from the brain to several parts of the body, such as the ear canal, larynx, esophagus, lungs, trachea, heart, and tongue. It provides information flow from these parts of the body to the brain. One of the systems it connects to is the gut and, more specifically, the stomach. When your gut is infected with harmful bacteria, it can hijack this nerve and send misleading signals to the brain. These signals can negatively impact your mood, weight, and decision-making.

Let us now move on to the next chapter, where you will learn how to get your body back to functioning at optimal capacity.

Chapter 5: How to Heal Your Body

"Be brave enough to heal yourself even if it hurts."

By Bianca Sparacino

The final stage of the road to recovery is understanding how to reverse the tremendous damage done to your gut. Crohn's disease is an illness that can haunt you for decades, and with each passing year, the damage to your gut gets worse and worse if it is left untreated.

This final step is about understanding how you can leverage the right biological processes to maximize the healing process. Diet is a major component of this process, so this is where we will begin.

The first thing to understand is that when you've eaten something, and the process of digestion begins, this has a tremendous impact on other bodily functions. All non-essential body processes are either put on hold or slowed down to prioritize energy allocation to the digestive process. Unfortunately, this can also mean that helpful processes such as cell repair, toxin removal, elimination of dead cells, and stem cells' production can also be halted.

With this in mind, it becomes obvious that your goal should be to reduce the amount of time your body spends on digesting food to maximize cell repair to the damage caused by Crohn's disease.

A diet consisting of sugar is counterproductive to this goal. This is because sugar gives a temporary boost of energy that gives you the illusion of strength, but it quickly fades after a while. This means you will have to eat again soon, and the digestion process will interfere with other bodily functions.

Therefore, your goal should be to structure meals that help lower the overall number of meals you will need in a day. This will give your body the much-needed moments of respite necessary for healing.

Carefully planned and executed intermittent fasting can help stem cell creation necessary to heal damaged regions of the body and improve blood sugar regulation.

Weston A. Price

I mentioned the name Weston A. Price at the beginning of the book, and now it's time I explained who he was and why his contributions are so significant. Most of the insights provided in this book are based on personal experiences. As much as I would like to take credit for the fantastic results, the truth is that I owe a lot of my success to the study of the literature written by a man who lived decades ago.

Weston A. Price was a Canadian doctor who lived in the late 19th century to mid 20th. He graduated from the University of Michigan and worked as a dentist. His profession allowed him to study the correlation between nutrition and dental and physical health in general.

His rise to fame was mainly based on the observation that many diseases found in westerners were not present in most nonwestern cultures. This led him to conclude that food's industrial production was stripping away many of the vital nutrients. The desire for higher quantity came at the cost of quality in nutrition. The west was able to surpass other societies in terms of wealth, but this came at a terrible cost compared to nonwestern societies. From Asia to Africa, many societies still based their entire diets on non-processed foods directly from farms. They did not use any chemicals to grow their foods, and nothing was taken through a factory to be stripped of essential nutrients.

Criticisms to the conclusions reached by professional skeptics such as William T Jarvis pointed out that many societies outside the West displayed signs of malnutrition, which would invalidate Price's ideas. This criticism is incorrect because malnutrition outside the West was due to a lack of sufficient food due to droughts and crop attacks by pests. The malnutrition was never the result of the type of foods they ate but rather the quantity.

Weston A. Price Dietary Advice

Doctor Price advised that food consumed should be as close to natural as possible, free of any processing. The closer you are to nature, the better off you are likely to be. Equally important to note is that even natural environments like rivers and oceans have become polluted by industrial waste. This means that you need to be careful about where the fish you eat comes from.

Dr. Price advised protein consumption from fish, eggs, poultry, lamb, and organ meats. Dr. Price also encouraged grass-fed meat to grain-fed meat, which is a topic that has been discussed in depth elsewhere.

Sweeteners should be used in moderation and should always be from natural, unprocessed sources. Raw honey, maple syrup, and date sugar are great substitutes.

Exercise and Crohn's Disease

A 2017 study published in the journal Clinical Experimental Gastroenterology revealed that exercise helps to mitigate many of the symptoms associated with Crohn's disease. In fact, people who exercise consistently have far fewer flare-ups of Crohn's disease than before they began exercising. Working out leads to improved energy levels, fewer instances of inflammation, and better mental health.

Unfortunately, Crohn's disease leads to physical limitations that make hardcore exercise routines effectively impossible. You will have to engage in mild exercises like aerobics, walking, cycling, dancing, swimming, and Pilates to get better and build your strength back up.

As I end this chapter, I will state that the road to healing is long and hard, but the results are worth it. So don't give up and keep fighting until you achieve your goals.

Conclusion

"As soon as healing takes place, go out and heal somebody else."

By Maya Angelou

In conclusion, I will recap the lessons in the chapters above. The first is that Crohn's disease is just like any other gut-related disease that results from infection. The only difference between them is which specific regions of the gut the infection attacks. The infection could be of a bacterial or fungal nature.

While genetic factors play a role in terms of risk, the infection is primarily caused by poor dieting choices or the use of antibiotics that kill good gut bacteria and cause an imbalance within the digestive system. Taking control of what goes into your body is the key to improving the quality of bacteria that resides in the gut.

Many of the symptoms associated with Crohn's disease can be quite embarrassing. Diarrhea, chronic abdominal pain, and blood in stool are not topics that one likes to reveal about themselves. I remember my struggle with talking about what I was going through. It may feel easier to hide your symptoms, but this is not a good idea. The longer you take before you start taking control of your condition, the greater the damage you will have to deal with later on. It's not just the physical consequences you have to worry about; the psychosocial and psychological toll of living in pain and shame can be pretty tough to deal with. If you need to talk to a therapist, then there is no shame in this.

It's also important to note that getting better requires sacrifice on your part. When you visit a restaurant with friends, you need to have the discipline to say no to eating food that you believe may not be safe for you. The dietary restrictions mentioned in the chapters above mean that you will have to rethink everything you can and cannot eat.

Sugar is very appealing, but you must cultivate the strength required to change how you live. I have found that the best way to achieve the best results is to find substitutes for the various foods which I previously liked but can no longer enjoy.

Thank You

Finally, thanks for taking the time to read this book. The information contained within doesn't simply come from intense research but, more importantly, from personal experience. You can trust the information contained within because I have gone through what you are going through now. I do not present theoretical abstractions but rather a personalized account of how I refused to accept defeat and chose to fight back.

I suffered for years with Crohn's disease before I finally found a solution to my problems. The lessons contained in this book didn't simply put an end to my suffering but also saved my life as well.

Note: It's easy to go through life ignoring a problem until it is too late. If you choose to ignore the damage inflicted by Crohn's disease to your gut, the results could be life-threatening. It's also tempting to blame other people for your problems, but this will lead you into a worse state than you were before.

I advise you to follow through with the advice provided in this book to the letter, and I promise that you will begin to see improvements in your life.

Thanks again, and I wish you the best of luck on your road to recovery.

Printed in Great Britain
by Amazon